AF578374

Secret nobody talks about masturbation

And how it destroys you

By

Renee R Tomas

table of content

Chapter one

What is Masturbation

In straightforward terms, masturbation includes contacting your privates (or other delicate regions) for sexual joy. In any case, masturbation is a mind-boggling subject and it's likewise one that is frequently not discussed.

Sorts of masturbation

Masturbation shifts from one individual to another and there isn't one sort of masturbation since everybody is unique. Masturbation can include any kind of sensual contacting or feeling. For instance, clitoral or areola excitement and butt-centric or vaginal infiltration are all considered sorts of masturbation.

Masturbation should be possible all alone or with another person. By the day's end, masturbation is simply one more kind of sex, so assuming that you're doing it with another person, it should be consensual. What we find exciting is profoundly individual, yet what's significant is that you feel good. Masturbation will frequently include climax (sexual peak), however, this isn't generally the situation.

Who strokes off

A new report showed that 72% of men and 42% of ladies stroked off in the previous year. What's more, there isn't only one kind of individual who jerks off. Individuals of various ages, foundations, and sexual inclinations make it happen.

Masturbation among ladies is progressively normal. While there used to be a touch of disgrace and mystery around female sexuality, not any longer. Young lady power has come into full power!

Masturbation isn't mandatory and you're not unusual if you would rather not play with yourself. Certain individuals want to jerk off, and that is absolutely fine also.

masturbation portrays a stage that virtually every youngster goes through. In any case, in light of the sacred text, as well as having seen the example of "self-delight" worked out again and again in the existence of such a large number of men, we consider this to be high contrast, good and bad issue. Our reasons are many creases, and logic merit a more inside and out treatment than this concise article will allow, yet they include:

Sex was imagined and planned by God Himself for the motivations behind multiplication and to communicate closeness and love between a couple. Masturbation obviously doesn't satisfy God's motivation for sex.

Sex isn't a need, but instead a longing. We needn't bother with sex to live and thrive and satisfy the reasons for which we were made. In his book At the Altar of Sexual Idolatry, Steve Gallagher recognizes that the sex drive tops in the 5-multi day time frame after the last delivery, yet disseminates from there on to a reasonable level. Sacred writing scolds us to starve the tissue. (Colossians 3:5, Romans 8:13, Ephesians 4:22)

An act of masturbation will in general make one physically free. Hitched people never again shift focus over to their mate only for sexual delight, and become less ready to give the stuff to fulfill and be fulfilled totally with their accomplice. A solitary individual has one less motivation to genuinely commit to the sort of responsibility required for a faithful marriage.

An act of masturbation contradicts the ideals of poise, a product of the Spirit. (Galatians 5:23) Jesus said "Whoever wants to come after Me, let him deny himself, and take up his cross, and follow Me. For whoever wants

to save his life will lose it, yet whoever loses his life for the good of I and the gospel's will save it." (Mark 8:34-35) Denying "self" incorporates opposing the compulsion to delight ourselves with the joy of masturbation.
It is for all intents and purposes difficult to jerk off without fantasizing. The people who differ are messing with themselves. Jesus said, "However I tell you that whoever takes a gander at a lady to desire for her has previously dedicated infidelity with her in his heart." (Matthew 5:28) Jesus' words rule out the dreams that feed desire and masturbation.

Masturbation in the Bible - What does the Bible say regarding Masturbation?

The Bible doesn't examine masturbation unequivocally or notice whether it is wrongdoing. In any case, there are a few refrains that have been deciphered to certainly be referring to masturbation. The sacred writing statement generally regularly connected with masturbation is the story of Onan in Genesis 38:9-10. Some make sense of this section for really intend that "spilling your seed" is a transgression. Albeit in the story, Onan pulled out from playing out his obligation to give a replacement to his late sibling.

One more scriptural statement some of the time utilized as a sign that masturbation is wrongdoing is Matthew 5:27-30. Jesus denounces having lecherous expectations and afterward says, "If your right-hand makes you sin, cut it off and discard it." While there is clearly a relationship between obscenity and masturbation, it is dubious that Jesus was referring to the specific sin of masturbation in this stanza.

CHAPTER two

Risks of masturbation

Masturbation is sex with evil spirits. It contaminates and obliterates your body, the sanctuary of the Holy Spirit

1 Cor 6:18-19 Flee from extramarital perversion. Each and every other sin a man commits is outside his body, yet he who sins physically sins against his own body. Do you not realize that your body is a sanctuary of the Holy Spirit who is in you, whom you have gotten from God? You are not your own

Masturbation - Sex with Demons

Masturbation is about contemplations and minds. It's the consequence of not projecting down minds and carrying contemplations to the acquiescence of Christ (2 Cor 10:5)

Satan can take care of our contemplations and minds into our psyches when he isn't in that frame of mind from good ways; a distant. At the point when you consider his ideas minds and voices, you wind up doing what he needs, jerking off; erring.

As you fantasize about his viewpoints and minds, evil spirits begin controlling your body, making you jerk off - you can't see them truly with your eyes however they are there

Today the adversary has concocted sex toys, and sex objects, to help masturbation, to take kill, and annihilate mankind totally. Sex toys are an industry of Satan.

Masturbation is a soul - an evil presence. This soul of murkiness doesn't come alone, it is joined by the soul of desire.

The soul of desire incorporates desire for eyes, the desire for tissue, and so on. One of the spirits takes individuals to porn and a wide range of extramarital perversion.
Sexual entertainment is fuel for masturbation.

Masturbation is a transgression that develops exceptionally quick into the habit - an extremely terrible fixation
Masturbation can result from generational revile, acquired from one age to another. Our folks and progenitors never let us know the transgressions they did, addictions and condemnations they were in, then, at that point, when we and our kids begin acquiring these condemnations, the vast majority of us fault God, others and see God in a terrible light.
Assuming that you are in masturbation or were, don't be amazed if your kids and grandkids are in masturbation as well.

Profound a couple is likewise a reason for masturbation. Profound a couple are of the whore realm which incorporates Jezebel, marine realm, and so forth

How DOES the SPIRIT OF MASTURBATION Respond?

Masturbation is a feeling of Satan whose work is to take kill and obliterate (John 10:10)

Masturbation debases and annihilates the sanctuary of the Lord - the body (1 Cor 6)

It obliterates the body that you can't satisfy your significant other or spouse nor be satisfied (1 Cor 7)

It obliterates the body of a man that a man can pass out sperms with simply an idea or creative mind - its one reason for untimely discharge.

Combined with the soul of desire, it makes an individual a creature - from your viewpoints, to how you act, what you see and need to see, wild longings and inclinations, and so forth - you become a creature

Masturbation causes stagnation with no leap forward

Each individual who jerks off watches porn and is engaged with any type of extramarital perversion is in life stagnation somehow.

Masturbation, erotic entertainment, and all types of extramarital perversion close entryways that in the event that you should be in point B you never move from point A however stale at point A.

At the point when the foe knows in the otherworldly domain that there is a forward leap or favors coming, he causes you to stroke off or be engaged with any type of extramarital perversion, and by that he has closed your gifts, forward leap, and so forth - he has taken. What's more, this is the greatest reason for stagnation in many individuals in the congregation today.

By utilizing the entryway of masturbation, the adversary can present to you any revile, hardship, and torture as he wills - he can take as he wills

Many individuals want marriage yet can't get it since masturbation porn and extramarital perversion has closed it from them

How masturbation kills marriage furtively

Chances are, your father never conversed with you about it while you were growing up.

In any case, it's an excruciating issue for the vast majority of Christian men out there. Single men, specifically, can't help thinking about what they ought to do until they get hitched. They might try and inquire, "Isn't it better to jerk off and fulfill my regular cravings in this manner as opposed to some — 'more clear' type of sexual sin

One of the difficulties in addressing these inquiries is that the mainstream world has been caught up with normalizing masturbation and scattering adverse results (however it truly isn't a fact that you will go visually impaired). A large number of us who have gone to instructors, even ministers, about our own masturbation propensities have been told, "Don't stress over that! That is typical." without a doubt the encounter of jerking off is exceptionally normal. Indeed, even children contact themselves and find the experience pleasurable. Numerous teenagers coincidentally find the experience again when it has become orgasmic and track down it both invigorating and startling simultaneously. That doesn't sin, yet ordinary interest.

The primary test to addressing these inquiries men pose is that the Bible never makes reference to the word masturbation. Without even a trace of an unmistakable order, we ought to be cautious that we don't stack fix judgment where God planned it. However, there are a few things that we ought to remember.

While the Bible isn't clear about masturbation, it is clear about an indecent dream. In Matthew 5:27-28, Jesus instructs that pondering another lady lewdly is infidelity. Assuming you're hoping to legitimize masturbation, you must get some information about when you do it. Carrying yourself to climax while pondering anybody to whom you are not hitched is, as indicated by Jesus, infidelity. Contemplating some sexual situation and accomplishing a climax to those considerations conditions you to what sex could be like. This is hazardous in that it sets up unreasonable assumptions about what sex with your significant other — or future spouse — ought to be like.

Rundown of how masturbation kills your marriage

1 low sex drive
2 difficulty
3 unfit to get fun with your accomplice
4. Hardships

Justifications for WHY MASTURBATION IS WRONG.

Loss of interest in marriage:

Most men that effectively practice the demonstration of masturbation will in time lose a taste for the establishment of marriage.

1.Death toll center:

The men that effectively jerk off will generally consider it more often than not. It is pretty much as terrible as per some clinicians, there are men who contemplate jerking off like clockwork making them lose center around the main things throughout everyday life. A man's contemplations should be overwhelmingly about his life's objectives, missions, and purposes.

Sensations of the feeling of inadequacy:

By and large, when men practice masturbation on a standard premise, they foster sensations of the feeling of inadequacy. They will more often than not imagine that they are not ordinary and at times they assume they are the only ones experiencing this habit. They think others are ordinary while they are not.

2.Late relationships:

They are typically late relationships among individuals who are dependent on rehearsing masturbation for quite a while. They find it hard to prepare themselves prepared and do not see a lot of need for it ethically. At times they fear the obligations that accompany marriage.

3.Unfortunate sexual dreams:

The vast majority who are associated with masturbation can't actually manage without fantasizing. This course of fantasizing could be as violent and unavoidable in the brain as it could get. This turns into an issue in marriage when a wedded man is laying down with his better half yet in his dreams he is really not seeing his significant other but rather different ladies.

4.The tissue is voracious:

Individuals engaged with masturbation sometimes find that the yearning for sexual fulfillment is unquenchable. Consequently, the most common way of looking for joy generally grounds such a person in the most corrupt acts of sexual invasion including requesting the administration of whores and escorts.

5 It bring sexual invasion into marriages

For a wedded man who was accustomed to jerking off before marriage, the debasement could proceed to the degree of him not having the option to be physically stimulated by his life partner. In this case, most men need to result to watching obscene movies and pictures while they have intercourse with their spouses any other way they can not persuade themselves to be stimulated.

6.Masturbation could prompt swinging in marriage:

The level of sexual invasion that outcomes from masturbation are called pleasure seeker parties when men who are not any more stirred by their accomplices go to the degree of participating in sex with other wedded couples. In any event, going to the degree of organizing bash parties for it.

7.Masturbation could prompt sexual fetishism:

Many young fellows approach taking women's clothing or drawing near to ladies' private effects to involve them as a demonstration of sexual delight. This is because of a long act of self-satisfaction through masturbation that presently searches for an all the more obvious gesture. This ordinarily happens to men that miss the mark on guts and strength to move toward a woman. It is a type of dependence.

8.Obscene fixation:

The vast majority who practice masturbation wind up becoming dependent on erotic entertainment since it gives mystery and it permits quicker interaction of imagination and discharge. The issue is that it becomes habit-forming sometime.

9.Masturbation prompts terrible sexual invasion:

Individuals who begin with masturbation have been viewed as trapped in an assault, sex with creatures, twistedness, sadomasochism, and other unfathomable invasions. This is on the grounds that the tissue can never be fulfilled. The dream and the quest for sexual fulfillment are interminable.

10..Masturbation prompts prostrate-related sicknesses:

A great many people who are effectively associated with masturbation get complexities in their later years, in light of various confusions they have with their wellbeing after the age of 40. It could not be guaranteed to prompt prostate disease for everyone, but rather it gives sufficient well-being worries to be concerned.

11.Self-centeredness and egocentrism in marriage:

An individual that is accustomed to fulfilling himself physically through masturbation keeps on doing that even after he is hitched. The spouse will be continually disappointed in light of the fact that the husband isn't accustomed to fulfilling others however himself.

12.Untimely discharge:

One of the primary issues in marriage for individuals who have been associated with masturbation is untimely discharge. Why that is an issue is that when a man experiences untimely discharge, the lady as a rule stays unsatisfied which could prompt complexities in the marriage.

13.Erectile brokenness:

Whenever somebody participates in masturbation sufficiently long, it arrives at a moment that you don't actually require an erection to discharge and once a man discharges he is fulfilled however in marriage this turns into an issue since erection is important to physically fulfill an accomplice. It is additionally essential for multiplication.

14.Sensations of Guilt and self-judgment:

One of the most over-the-top horrendous outcomes of masturbation is that a great many people who participate in it experience sensations of culpability and self-judgment consistently, which is likewise a sign to us that carrying on with an existence of masturbation isn't regular.

15.Melancholy and agony:

Masturbation frequently brings about sensations of melancholy and agony. The vast majority who are associated with masturbation become testy and shut in light of the fact that they fear imparting their experience to individuals in view of the apprehension about judgment and being misconstrued.

Powerlessness to fabricate solid relationship with the other gender:

A great many people who are associated with masturbation are so used to living inside themselves, that they agree with themselves that they frequently don't have the foggiest idea how to fabricate the muddled relationship with the other gender. In a relationship, you want to continually figure out what the other individual's advantage is.

This could prompt men to avoid the chance to wed or even to separate after marriage.

CHAPTER 3

5Biblical Ways to Overcome Masturbation

Off-kilter or not, as Christians, this is a point we can't disregard. Our houses of worship and local area circles are loaded up with individuals who quietly battle with this wrongdoing, excessively humiliated to look for the assistance they with wanting to find.

Maybe you are somebody who battles with masturbation. Or then again maybe you do not know why this is an enticement for individuals however might want to be somebody others can trust and get counsel from. One way or another, the following are five functional pointers that will assist Christians with beating the wrongdoing of masturbation.

1. Realize the Bible Actually Does Condemn Masturbation

You've presumably heard that "masturbation" is found no place in Scripture, which is

totally obvious. In this manner when the vast majority make sense of why masturbation is a transgression, they center around the lascivious contemplations and goals that are quite often connected with self-joy.
However, the grounds that the Bible doesn't straightforwardly denounce masturbation doesn't mean it has not been prohibited in a roundabout way. Regularly creators in the Bible talk in classes as opposed to in particulars. So as opposed to posting each conceivable sexual demonstration that could be evil, the Bible gives us general limits within which we are to remain.

To the wedded 1 Corinthians 7:5 states, "Don't deny each other with the exception of maybe by common assent and for a period, so you might dedicate yourselves to petition. Then meet up again so Satan won't entice you on account of your absence of poise." To the single 1 Corinthians 7:9 makes sense, "Yet on the off chance that they have no control over themselves, they ought to wed, for it is smarter to wed than to get overwhelmed with emotion."

These two refrains give us one sexual class for both the wedded and the single that incorporates all approved sexual demonstrations: All sexual action should incorporate the actual presence of your companion.

Masturbation is by implication denounced through what is explicitly excused. Notice Paul says that assuming you are hitched and play out a sexual demonstration away from your mate, you have tumbled to Satan's enticement due to your absence of restraint. Assuming that you are single and play out any sexual demonstration (since you don't have a life partner), here again, Paul says you are demonstrating the way that you have zero control over yourself since you are enjoying sexual movement implied for marriage alone.

Since masturbation is done away from your life partner, the Bible arranges it as transgression. You can't quit jerking off on the off chance that you are not persuaded it is corrupt. Subsequently, the most important phase in halting this transgression is to be solidly persuaded that the Bible censures this demonstration.

(For a more profound glance at what the Bible says regarding masturbation, read the article, "Does the Bible Say Masturbation Is Sin?)

2. Try not to Use Weird Mental Tactics to Justify This Sin

The demonstration of masturbation generally begins in the psyche. Regardless of whether you've never heard the scriptural rationale communicated in point 1, we as a whole know subliminally masturbation is wrongdoing. To get around this, individuals frequently utilize odd contentions in their minds to legitimize why they are enjoying self-delight.

I've conversed with single individuals who have figured out how to stroke off while "contemplating nothing," hence they believe they are not craving, which in their brains makes self-delight OK. I've known about individuals who legitimize masturbation by expressing it helps them not commit more awful sexual sins like taking a gander at pornography or having early sex. I know wedded men who feel that for however long they are contemplating their significant other when they jerk off, then it is okay in God's eyes.

There are innumerable peculiar contentions we could attempt to use to legitimize masturbation. Be that as it may, according to God, sin will be sin. Keep it straightforward and simply comply with face-esteem your still, small voice, the Spirit's driving, and the Bible's guidelines.

3. Look Ahead to the Reward

To defeat any enticement, we want to oppose insidiously as well as seek after what is great. Romans 12:21 says, "Don't be overwhelmed by evil, yet conquer evil with great."

Assuming you are single and want to conquer masturbation, you need to solidly accept that your restraint and benevolence currently will bring about more noteworthy delight from here on out. You should figure out how to oppose the enticement as well as to seek after the joy that stems from satisfying God.

Moreover, masturbation will reduce your thoroughly enjoying sex once you get hitched. The more you oppose sexual allurement now, the more noteworthy your sexual encounters with your future mate will be later. Also, more than that, the more you oppose sin as a general rule, the more noteworthy your experience of God will be.

4. Don't Underemphasize the Practical Stuff

Is it safe to say that you are more enticed to stroke off late around evening time? Quit remaining up so late. Do R-evaluated films plant seeds of sexual sin in you that feed your evil nature? Quit watching these kinds of films. Does going to the ocean side or the rec center reason you to see the other gender in a meager dress? Try not to go to these spots any longer.

Distinguish any triggers and cut them out. Battling masturbation is an otherworldly fight, however, don't underrate the down-to-earth stuff by the same token.

5. Recall Who You Are in Christ

The course of blessing is straightforwardly attached to our ability to embrace the impacts the gospel has had on us. At the point when we become a Christian, we are made into another creation with wants to satisfy God (2 Corinthians 5:14-21). We should now use whatever might remain of our lives to figure out how to embrace our new recognize and dismiss our old nature.

If you have any desire to beat the compulsion to stroke off, you should trust your Bible over your sentiments. Teach reality to yourself, "I'm another creation in Christ. I would rather not sin like this. I need to satisfy God now." The more profoundly you accept that you are a renewed individual who desires virtue as opposed to wantonness, the more your activities will start to change.

In the event that you are a Christian, you are another creation. Presently you simply have to trust it and live from this reality.

A Guide to Self-Control against masturbating

1. Never contact the personal pieces of your body besides during ordinary latrine processes.
2. Abstain from being distant from everyone else however much as could be expected. Track down the great organization and remain in this great organization.
3. In the event that you are related to different people having this equivalent issue, YOU MUST BREAK OFF THEIR FRIENDSHIP. Never partner with others having a similar shortcoming. Try not to assume that you two will stop together, you won't ever will. You should move away from individuals of that sort. Just to be in their presence will keep your concern premier to

you. The issue should be removed From YOUR MIND for that is where it truly exists. Your psyche should be on other and more healthy things.

4. At the point when you wash, don't respect yourself in a mirror. Never stay in the shower more than five or six minutes - - sufficiently lengthy to wash and dry and dress AND THEN GET OUT OF THE BATHROOM into a room where you will have some individual from your family present.

5. At the point when in bed, assuming that is where you have your concern generally, dress for the evening so safely that you can only with significant effort contact your fundamental parts, thus that it would be troublesome and tedious for you to take off those garments. When you began to take off defensive attire you would have adequately controlled your reasoning that the enticement would leave you.

6. On the off chance that the enticement appears to be overwhelming while you are sleeping, GET OUT OF BED AND GO INTO THE KITCHEN AND FIX YOURSELF A SNACK, regardless of whether it is around midnight, and regardless of whether you are not eager, and in spite of your apprehensions about putting on weight. The reason behind this idea is that you GET YOUR MIND ON SOMETHING ELSE. You are the subject of your viewpoints, in a manner of speaking.

7. Never read explicit material. Never read about your concern. Keep it out of your psyche. Keep in mind - - "Initial an idea, then, at that point, a demonstration." The idea design should be changed. You should not permit this issue to stay with you. At the point when that's what you achieve, you before long will be liberated from the demonstration.

8. Put healthy contemplations into your psyche consistently. Peruse great books - - Church books - - Scriptures - - Sermons of the Brethern [sic, Cistern too?]. Make a day-to-day propensity for perusing something like one section of Scripture, ideally from one of the four Gospels in the New Testament, or the Book of Mormon. The four Gospels - - Matthew, Mark, Luke, and John - - above whatever else in the Bible can be useful in light of their elevating characteristics.

9. Supplicate. However, when you ask, don't supplicate about this issue, for that will more often than not keep [it] to you like never before. Appeal to God for confidence, petition God for comprehension of the Scriptures, petition God for the Missionaries, the General Authorities, your companions, and your families, BUT KEEP THE PROBLEM OUT OF YOUR MIND BY NOT MENTIONING IT EVER - - NOT IN CONVERSATION WITH OTHERS, NOT

IN YOUR PRAYERS. KEEP IT _OUT_ of your psyche!

The disposition of an individual toward his concern has an influence [sic] on the fact that it is so natural to survive. It is fundamental that a strong responsibility is made to control the propensity. As an individual grasps his explanations behind the way of behaving and is delicate to the circumstances or circumstances that might set off a craving for the demonstration, he fosters the ability to control it.

We are instructed that our bodies are sanctuaries of God, and are to be spotless so the Holy Ghost might stay inside us. Masturbation is a corrupt propensity that denies one of the Spirit and makes culpability and close-to-home pressure. It isn't genuinely hurtful except if drilled to the limit. A propensity is absolutely egotistical, and cryptic, and not the slightest bit communicates the legitimate utilization of the procreative power given to man to satisfy timeless motivations. It hence isolates an individual from God and losses the gospel plan.

This self-satisfying action will make one lose his self-esteem declaration becomes feeble, and preacher work and other Church reasons for living become oppressive contributions.

To help in arranging a successful program to defeat the issue orientation is given on how the regenerative organs in a young fellow capability.

The testicles in your body are persistently delivering many millions of the _vas deferens_ to a spot called the _ampulla_ where they are blended in with liquids from two membranous pockets called _seminal vesicles_ and the _prostate gland_.

It is typical for the vesicles to be exhausted incidentally around evening time during the discharging of coming from the central sensory system. Frequently a sensual dream is competent simultaneously and is a piece of this typical interaction. Rather than a course, the regenerative framework is working at a more fast speed, attempting to stay aware of the deficiency of semen. At the point when he stops the propensity, the body will keep on delivering at his expanded rate.

As one meets with his Priesthood Leader, a program for conquering masturbation can be executed utilizing some of t Remember it is fundamental that a standard report program is settled on, so progress can be perceived and disappointments got and killed.

Suggestions

1. Implore day to day, request the gifts of the Spirit, what will fortify you against enticement. Implore intensely and not boor when the allurements are the most grounded.
2. Follow a program of incredible day-to-day work out. The activities lessen close-to-home pressure and gloom and are totally essential to the arrangement of this issue. Twofold your active work when you feel pressure expanding.
3. At the point when the compulsion to jerk off serious areas of strength for is, _STOP_ to those contemplations as uproariously as you could to you and afterward at any point discuss a prechosen Scripture or sing a persuasive song. It is essential to dismiss your considerations from the self-centered need to enjoy.
4. Put forth objectives of restraint, start with a day, then seven days, month, or year lastly focus on at absolutely no point ever doing it in the future. Until you concede to _never

again_ you will constantly be available to allurement.

5. Change in conduct and demeanor is most handily accomplished through a changed mental self-view. Invest energy consistently envisioning major areas of strength for yourself in charge, effectively conquering enticing circumstances.

6. Start to work day to day on a personal growth program. Relate this intention to further developing your Church administration, to working on your associations with your family, God, and others. Endeavor to improve your assets and gifts.

7. Be active and cordial. Drive yourself to accompany others and figure out how to appreciate functioning and conversing with them. Use standards of creating companionships found in books like _How to Win Friends and Influence People_ by Dale Carnegie.

8. Know about circumstances that push down you or that make you feel desolate, exhausted, baffled, or deterred. These profound states can set off the craving to stroke off as a method of break. Plan ahead of time to counter these low periods through different exercises, for example, perusing a book, visiting a companion, accomplishing something athletic, and so on.

9. Make a pocket schedule for a month on a little card. Convey it with you, yet show it to nobody. In the event that you have a slip by of discretion, variety the day dark. Your objective will be to have _no dark days_. The schedule turns into major areas of strength for a sign of poise and ought to be taken a gander at when you are enticed to add another dark day. Keep your schedule up until you have no less than three clear months.

10. A cautious report will show you have had the issue at specific times and under specific

circumstances. Attempt and review, exhaustively, what your specific times and conditions were. Now that you comprehend how it works out, plan to break the example through counter exercises.

11. In the field of psychotherapy, there is an exceptionally viable strategy called _aversion therapy_. At the point when we partner or consider something extremely tacky with something which has been pleasurable, however unwanted, the disagreeable idea and feeling will start to counteract what was pleasurable. Assuming you partner something extremely tacky with your deficiency of restraint it will assist you with halting the demonstration. For instance, on the off chance that you are enticed to stroke off, consider washing in a tub of worms, and eating a few of them as you do the demonstration.

12. During your toileting and shower exercises leave the washroom entryway or

shower drapery part of the way open, to deter being distant from everyone else in absolute security. Clean up.

13. Emerge quickly in the mornings. Try not to lie in bed alert, regardless of what season of the day it is. Get up and follow through with something. Begin every day with energetic action.

14. Keep your bladder vacant. Shun drank a lot of liquids prior to resigning.

15. Lessen how many flavors and fixings are in your food. Eat as softly as conceivable around evening time.

16. Wear night robes that are challenging to open, yet free and not restricting.

17. Keep away from individuals, circumstances, pictures, or perusing materials that could make sexual fervor.

18. It is at times supportive to have an actual item to use in beating this issue. A Book of Mormon, solidly held close by, even in bed

around evening time has demonstrated support in outrageous cases.

19. In exceptionally extreme cases it very well might be important to attach a hand to the bed outline with a tie together so that the propensity for stroking off in a semi-rest condition can be broken. This can likewise be achieved by wearing a few layers of dress which would be hard to eliminate while drowsy.

20. Set up a prize framework for your triumphs. It doesn't need to be a major prize. A quarter in a container each time you survive or arrive at an objective. Spend it on something which delights you and will be a proceeding with an indication of your advancement.

21. Try not to allow yourself to get back to any past propensity or disposition designs that were a contributor to your concern. _Satan Never Gives Up_. Be smoothly and unhesitatingly wary. Keep a positive mental

disposition. You can win this battle! The delight and strength you will feel when you truly do will provide for what seems like forever with a brilliant and otherworldly shine of fulfillment and satisfaction.

Yours eternity in Christ,

www.ingramcontent.com/pod-product-compliance
Lightning Source LLC
LaVergne TN
LVHW020524160826
845677LV00015B/3893

* 9 7 9 8 8 4 8 1 5 1 3 3 6 *